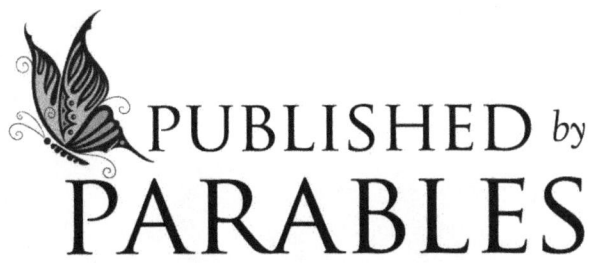

# Can You See The Stress?
## I Do Now!

## Gail Comminie

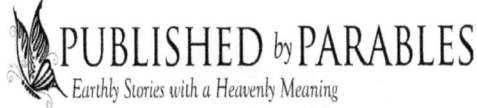
PUBLISHED by PARABLES
*Earthly Stories with a Heavenly Meaning*

Can You See The Stress?  I Do Now!
Gail Comminie


Copyright © Gail Comminie

*Published By Parables*
August, 2018

All Rights Reserved. No part of this book may be reproduced or utilized in any form or by any means, electronic or mechanical, including photocopying, recording, or by any information storage and retrieval system, without permission in writing from the author.

Unless otherwise specified Scripture quotations are taken from the authorized version of the King James Bible.

    ISBN 978-1-945698-68-2
    Printed in the United States of America

Readers should be aware that Internet Web sites offered as citations and/or sources for further information may have been changed or disappeared between the time this was written and when it is read.

# Can You See The Stress?
## I Do Now!

## Gail Comminie

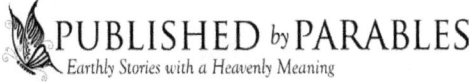
Earthly Stories with a Heavenly Meaning

# GAIL COMMINIE

# DEDICATION

This Book is how my life changed after suffering three strokes. I was living a life under so much stress and never realized it or the danger that comes with it. October 28, 2013 was the turning point in my life. Everything changed that day. I had to make some changes that affected me financially, mentally and physically. When life throws you a curve ball what do you do?

I am dedicating this book to my husband
Rev. Joseph Comminie Jr.

Also I am dedicating this book in the memory of
my parents
Jessel Sr. and Eunice Samuel Smith,
my brother, Jessel Smith Jr. and
my in-laws
Joseph Sr. and Leanne Favorite Comminie.

# INTRODUCTION:

October 28, 2013, December 15, 2013 and January 2014, I suffered a stroke. Three stroke. The second stroke left me in a wheelchair and with a speech impairment. My Neurologist told me and my husband, because of the location and size of the stroke, I should have been permanently paralyzed or dead. But I am here. Three Strokes and I live, recovered, able to tell my story.

What is a stroke? Deuteronomy 28:61, "also every sickness and every stroke which is not in the book of this law, Jehovah doth cause them to go up unto thee till thou art destroyed."

A Stroke, also call CVA, cerebrovascular accident, is damage to the brain from interruption of its blood supply. A stroke is a "brain attack". It can happen to anyone at any time.

My experience, working in the medical field, is what saved my life. I knew the warning signs!!

# Chapter 1:
## "Who am I"

Psalm 139:13-16, "For you formed my inward parts, you knitted me together in my mother's womb. I praise you, for I am fearfully and wonderfully made. Wonderful are your works, my soul knows it very well, My frame was not hidden from you, when I was being made in secret, in intricately woven in the depths on earth, Your eyes saw my unformed substances; in your book were written, every one of them, the days that were formed for me, when as yet there was none of them."

I am a Child of God. God is my first love. I give Thanks to God that He has brought me through a difficult time in my life. I am grateful that He has chosen me to be a testimony and to tell my story how He has brought me to help someone else.

My birth name is Gail Marie Smith. I was born, February 13, 1953, the third child of Jessel Sr. and Eunice Smith. My siblings are Terry, Linda, Monna, Yolanda, Jessel Jr., Kemon and Donald Smith. I was born and raise in Edgard, Louisiana.

Even though I come from a large family, I always

felt like I was a outcast. What I mean is, my siblings to me have always looked at me or made me feel that I was less than them. I never felt like I belonged. I was never a person who expressed herself or really said how I feel or felt about things. I know that my parents loved me, but I never felt they understood me or understand the pain that was inside of me. There were eight children and I guess there was not time to spend with one to really understand or know what the other children were going through. I grew up feeling rejected, looked down on by my siblings, who I loved very much. Why the indifference toward me? I really would like to know. This feeling of rejection, I believe has affected me as I grew up and followed me into my adult life.

Sibling is mentioned throughout the Bible, Old and New Testament. Some of the most famous siblings we find are Cain and Abel, (Genesis 4:1-8). Cain killed Abel out of jealously. Jacob and Esau. (Genesis 25:18-27). They were at odd from the time they were in the womb and into adulthood. Joseph and eleven brothers (Genesis 37). His brothers sold him into slavery in Egypt. Mary and Martha, Lazarus (John 11:1) Their story contain a disagreement between them.

Love among sibling should be a natural thing. The Bible commands we should love one another in the family of God.

Romans 12:10, "Love one another with brotherly affection."

We are to love one another as it reflects the love of Christ. We are to be kind to each other, treat those in our family and around us the way we want to be treated. Love is very important and is needed, especially in the family is which we are born. Family is the first place and the first people we learn to love and learn the meaning of. My family grew up in the Church. We were brought up in the Catholic Faith by our Mother. My Grandfather was Rev. Landry Smith, a Baptist Minister. As we grew older and studied the Bible more, we learned that we are to love God first and that family is second to God.

Scripture: Ephesians 4:32, "be kind to one another, tenderhearted, forgiving one another, as God in Christ forgave you." Roman 14:10-12, "Why do you pass judgement on your brother. Or you, why do you despise your brother? For we will all stand before the judgement seat of God, for it is written, "As I live says the Lord, every knee shall bow to me, and every tongue shall confess to God". So then each of us will give an account of himself to God."

1 Corinthians 13:4-7, "Love is patient and kind; love does not envy or boast; it's not arrogant or rude, It does not insist on its own way; it is not irritable, or resentful; it does not rejoice at wrongdoing, but rejoices with the truth. Love bears all things, believes all things, hopes all things, endures all things."

As I grew, my imagination grew. I was always dreaming of ways to get even with people I thought were against me. I was always writing short stories and plays. I don't know where that was coming from. I have always loved writing and used it as a way to escape. I always felt that my siblings treated me as if I was strange, less and different. It hurt and somehow I was withdrawn. I kept to myself, in my own little world/corner and just let my imagination take over in my writing.

As a child/teenage, was I depressed or stressed? I can't answer that because that was never talked about or mentioned in my family. Maybe if someone had noticed, I could have gotten help.

My mother would always say to my Grandmother, "I don't know what wrong with that girl. She always keep to herself, never say much, but always thinking of ways to get in trouble. I don't know how she think of these things." I heard my Grandmother, Estella Samuel, say to her one day, "You know still water runs deep. What I mean is that, She is quiet and keep to herself, but that child is going places."

I grew up in Edgard, Louisiana. Edgard is a very close knit, family oriented community. It is a community where everybody knows everybody, There is not much here that happens that goes unnoticed. I love Edgard. I have traveled to other places, but there is no place like Edgard.

Growing up in the River Parishes, I have many memories, good and bad. As a child I remember playing in the quarters with my siblings and cousins. We climbed trees, played balls, jumped rope, picked berries and pecans, and played hide and seek. We never had cell phones, who ever heard of that! As a kid we would tie two cans to a string, that was our phone. Inside all day playing video games, no way!! We had to go outside. If your family had a phone, that meant you were fortunate. If you had a television, that was a Blessing. I remember we walked everywhere. If we fought, we fought with our hands and by the end of the day, it was all over with. I don't remember anyone dying because of a disagreement. As a child, we were never in adult conversation or around adults when they were talking. As a child, I remember we respected our elders. If they said you did something, you did it. You would probably get a whipping from them and one when you get home. Never pass on an adult/elder without speaking, don't cuss or talk back. When I was a child the whole village raised a child. If your Mom worked, then one neighbor had everybody's children. You ate what they ate and you had better obey!! Times have changed!!!

GAIL COMMINIE

## Chapter 2:
## "War Against The Family"

Today, we see war against the family. Modern pop culture is robbing our children of their innocence. There is random violence, filthy language and elicit sex. In spite of this brain washing, I believe that we can still win the war being waged against the family. The typical American family wasn't very different from that of today's family. There was no second or third automobile. There was no entertainment system, no cell phone. Some had a television and those who did, had only one or two stations.

There was no drug problem, there was no rampant sex, there was not a huge number of broken homes, there was no violence and crime in school. Why are we so stressed out? Can You See The Stress? I Do Now!

Fathers in my time, worked long and hard to make a living and put food on the table. In my time, Mom stayed home, taking care of the children and the home.

In my time, our entertainment was eating a cold watermelon on a warm day or making ice cream. Do you remember playing chute and ladder, monopoly, checkers, jump rope, marbles, ball, or hide and seek? Do you remember playing outdoors, not parked in front of the TV, or the computer, or playstation or on the cell phone?

In my time, my family had family time. We ate together. Family meals meant family time. It was the time when everyone got to tell about their day. It was at the dinner table, report cards were presented and discussed. It was at the dinner table, we would talk. Now today, everybody eat when they want, what they want, where they want, just not together.

Our parents showed us love. Love was not showering us with money or things, but by giving us time. We had chores and we earned or worked for what we wanted. We are stressed out, trying to please our children.

For many, the children run the home. Parents are afraid of their children. It is hard to tell who is the child and who are the adults. Children have their own rules, they get what they want and do as they please.

My parents read to us and my Grandmother used to sit on the porch and tell us stories. This is how we learned of our families' histories.

When it came to television program, it was something the whole family could watch.

Well those days are gone. It looks like we are so caught up on self and getting something for nothing. No more of that family value. Again, Why are we so stressed out? Can You See The Stress? I Do Now!

Today, the media plays a big role, a big responsibility in the war against the family. The media promotes, drugs, violence, gambling, adultery and sex. If you listen to the music our kids listen to, it is all sex, gang violence, language, disrespect, crime, killing, etc.... We live in a time of corrupt entertainment. Soap opera is about sex, murder and family betrayal. The cartoon shows are the same. The commercial is about everything and anything. **NOTHING IS SACRED!!! Can You See The Stress? I Do Now!**

Our children see and hear all of this and they are having a hard time, a great difficulty evaluating what is good and what is bad. This is where we as parents have to step in.

This war against the family isn't new. In fact it has been around since the very first family was formed on earth—the family consisting of Adam, Eve, Cain and Abel. They had no television, no magazine, no movies to seduce them. Still Adam and Eve sinned. Still, Cain murdered Abel (Genesis 4:8-9).

Genesis 4:8-9, "Cain spoke to Abel his brother, And when they were in the field, Cain rose up against his brother Abel and killed him. Then the Lord said to Cain, "Where is Abel your brother? He said, "I do not know; am I my brother's keeper?"

In the war against the family, Human nature is a constant factor. Jesus Christ said that human nature is a mix of human good and evil.

Luke 11:13, " If you then being evil, know how to give good gifts to your children, how much more shall your Heavenly Father give the Holy Spirit those who ask Him?"

The evil part of our human nature didn't come from God.

Genesis 1:31, "God saw all that he made, and it

was very good. And the evening and the morning was the sixth day".

Because we are created with the freedom of choice, we often choose evil because it appears more appealing to us.

Ephesians 2:1-3, " And you were dead in your trespasses and sins, In which you formerly walked according to the course of this world, according to the princes of the power of the air, of the so spirit that is now working in the sons of disobedience. Among them we too all formerly lived in the lusts of our flesh and of the mind, and were by nature children of wrath, even at the rest."

Another factor for the war against family is Satan the devil—a major role. The Bible refers to him as "the god of this age"

2 Corinthians 4:4, "In whose case the god of this world has blinded the minds of the unbelieving, that they might not see the light of the gospel of the glory of Christ, who is the image of God."

He is the world's unseen ruler at this time. This evil is out to destroy the family, out to destroy mankind.

1 Peter 5:8, "Be of sober spirit, be on the alert. Your adversary, the devil, prowls about like a roaring lion, seeking someone to devour".

We live in a world where everybody is fighting for their rights to do wrong.

If Satan can't influence us to kill one another through warfare, violence and crime, he'll make us miserable in any way he can, including the destruction of marriage and family. The evidence of this shows he has been remarkably successful. Our own selfish nature, wants and cravings play right into his hand. Again, why are we so stressed out? Can You See The Stress? I Do Now!

To create the best family environment, my advice is (1) put God first (2) Love your children (3) Show a genuine interest.

GAIL COMMINIE

## Chapter 3: "Marriage and Motherhood"

Ephesians 5:25, "for husband, this means love your wives, just as Christ loved the church. He gave up his life for her."

Genesis 2:24, "therefore a man shall leave his father and mother and hold fast to his wife, and they shall become one flesh."

I attended Second Ward Elementary School and Second Ward High School. I loved high school. I was very active. I loved baseball, gymnastic and was on the school dance team, Second Ward High School Eaglerettes. My best friends were Edna Haydel and Mary Nell Kelly. My favorite subject was Creative Writing and Drama. It was in High School that I discovered that I had a talent for writing and doing short plays. Even though I was good at it, I was never encouraged to pursue it as a career. It was September 1989 when I met Angela Thompson, Editor for Times Picayune, at a function at my church, that I was offered the chance to write, to put my skill/talent, my love for writing to work. I was offered the job of doing a article about the people/residents of the West Bank of St. John Parish. I accepted it and it was a very rewarding experience. I loved meeting the people, attending function and getting to know the many contributions and accomplishments of the people of Edgard, Louisiana and the West Bank of St. John Parish. The people/residents loved it. They loved and looked forward to my column every week. It kept them up on what was happening and the news and accomplishments of the residents. I was known as "River Road Rambling".

My husband and I also have written many plays and skits for our church, Greater New St. Peter Baptist Church. Our skits and plays has been performed in Churches in the community, throughout the Tri-Parish and in New Orleans. Our favorite skit we wrote and produced is "Look How far He Has Brought Me From". God has brought us from the bottom of a slave ship all the way to the White House.

The other that became famous is, "Jesus Last Words". This skit was preformed every Palm Sunday and it drew many to Church and many to Christ.

Unfortunately, my job as "River Road Rambling" ended January 2018. Every now and them I might be asked to do a feature story, which is not very often. That was a happy time for me. I was never stressed out, because I was doing what I love to do, "write".

I graduated from Second Ward High School, May 24, 1971. That same month, May 1, 1971, I married my high school sweetheart, Joseph Comminie Jr.

I was 18 and pregnant with my first child. I was married and in love and happy. I was only 18 and had a lot to learn. Yes, I was happy and excited and also scared. I was no longer under my parents' roof. Suddenly I am an adult and have adult responsibility. Married at 18 and didn't know anything about keeping a house or cleaning. Married and don't know anything about cooking. I don't even know how long to boil a egg or cook grits. If the show "Worst Cook" was aired in my time, I could have been the spokesperson for the show. For the first few weeks, it was living on love, but soon your stomach starts to groan for some home cooking. So I began cookng lesson from my sister-in-law Myrtis Young and my husband. My marriage was great at first. Joseph made me felt like I was a Queen. The love of his life. There was nothing he would not do for his queen. It was not long that Joseph began to change. I felt like I was walking on eggs. I no longer felt like his queen, but his punching bag and the verbal abuse was there also. The abuse, physical and mental, was so constant. I felt so ashamed. I had no one to talk to or nowhere to turn. I was not allowed to talk back or express myself. Battered, ashamed, withdrawn, tired and afraid. Where was God? My self esteem was so low. Black eyes and bruises, I had to hide. To the outside world, it looked like we were the perfect family, but behind closed door, I was a prisoner. It was his way or no way. He was in control. So many days and night I cried. The abuse went on for years. My self worth began to crumble. Soon I was turning to food to ease the pain and the weight began to add on. Food was my escape, my crutch. I even questioned my ability to be a loving wife, mother and if God loved me. On the outside we looked together, a happy couple and family. My husband appeared spiritually mature. He prayed eloquent prayer, went to school for Theology at Union Baptist College, New Orleans, Louisiana. He knew the Bible, could quote Scripture, explained Scripture, taught Sunday School and Bible Classes. He even counseled couples for Marriage, even performed marriage and baptized. He was and is very active in the Church. But behind closed doors, things weren't fine. I was unable to predict when the switch would flip on Joseph's anger. I walked on eggshell, Without warning, I'd suddenly become the object of his anger, uncontrolled, frightening rage. Because our situation was so intense, I was in constant prayer and conversation with God. I was looking for Scripture to find direction and connection to my Savior. "Can you see the stress? I Do Now!!

My first born, Tammy Lynette, was born, October 25, 1971. I had no idea what to do with a child, Thank God for my Mother-in-Law, Leanne Comminie and my mother for their support. Tammy cried a lot, She was spoiled and the apple of her Daddy's eye. He loved that little girl and everything he did was because of her, his first born. When she was 10, she was hit by a school bus while riding her bike. She had damage to her right leg. It was an accident. The bus driver did not see her passing in front of the bus. Tammy attended West St. John Elementary School and West St, John High School. She graduated June 3, 1989. She was baptized at the Gretaer New St. Peter Church, November 1980. Tammy married Leonard Gullage on February 14,

1993   Together they have three children, Anastasia, Leonard Jr., and Larenz and one grandchild, Aubrie Lynette Gullage

Unfortunately her husband, Leonard, is in prison. That is another time in my life that the stress and tension was great. I will tell you about that time a little later.

Tammy is a hard working person, a good mother. Her children and grandchild are the first and most important things in her life. She is quiet, but you don't want to cross her. I pray everyday for my child. Thanks to God for her strength and determination to be the best Mother and role model for children.

My second child, Shantel Renee, was born March 18, 1974 at Charity Hospital, New Orleans. She was baptized at the Greater New St. Baptist Church, January 1981. Shantel was a beautiful baby. She was a quick learner. She was a child who just had to know and need an answer for everything. She was very gifted. At the age of three, she was already reading, writing and learning her numbers. We had to find things for her to do just to keep her from getting bored.

Shantel graduated from West St. John High School, as Valedictorian, May 23, 1992. She graduated Cum Laude with a degree in Political Science and History from Louisiana Tech University, August 1995, She graduated with a Doctor of Jurisprudence from Loyola University New Orleans School of Law in December 2000.

She also graduated with a Master of Science in Curriculum and Instruction from Western Governors University, April 2013. She received her Master

Endorsement in Education Leadership from Western Governors University, April 2014.

Shantel is married to Shannon Pierrre Octave. They have two son, Shannon Jr. and Shayler Octave.

My third child is Joseph "JJ" Comminie III. He was born August 21, 1980 at Charity Hospital New Orleans. He was baptized at the Greater New St. Peter Baptist Church, July 6, 1986. JJ is my first son. He was a a very beautiful and handsome little boy. He was very spoiled. JJ was always very playful and very friendly. He likes to joke around and love family. He also attended West St. John High School and he graduated May 19, 1999. JJ is married to Mtisa Comminie. They have one child together, Jeremiah, and three from Mtisa's previous relationships, Randall and Syan Clark and Danasha Harris, and two grandchildren, Jaceon and Jason Deberry.

My fourth Child is Jamaal Anthony. Jamaal was born June 12, 1983 at Thibodaux Hospital. He was baptized at the Greater New St. Peter Baptist Church, September 4, 1988. Jamaal was also a beautiful baby boy. Jamaal is a mischievous child. He likes to joke around and get into things. I could never take him seriously. You never know when he was joking or telling the truth. With Jamaal you just had to take your chances. Jamaal graduated from West St. John High School, May 19, 2001. He also graduated ITT Technical Institution, July 26, 2003 with a Associate Degree.

He married Ranada Smith Comminie, November 24, 2007. They have two son, Jamaal Jr. and Ja'Quan Comminie.

# Chapter 4:
## "My Parents"
## The loss of parents can be so intense and overwhelming.

Psalm 23, 4, "Yea, though I walk through the valley of the shadow of death, I will fear no evil; for You are with me; Your rod and Your staff, they comfort me." Isaiah 41:10, Fear not, for I am with you; be not dismayed, for I am your God. I will strengthen you, yes, I will help you, I will uphold you with My righteous right hand.'

My Dad Jessel and my Mom Eunice were the two people in my life that have influence me the most. My Mom Eunice was born on May 12, 1936, the mother of eight children. She is the one that kept the family together. My Mother is the one that made sure she had a meal on the table, kept clothes on our back, made sure we were educated and attended church. My most precious memories of Mother is that of Christmas 1988. It was the last Christmas I spent with my mother, Eunice Samuel Smith. She died the day after that year.

Christmas was always my mother's favorite time of the year. My memories of Christmases with my mother are happy ones. Weeks before the holiday, she cooked, baked, decorated and shopped. On Christmas, my mother, Dad, four brothers, three sisters and I would gather together to exchange gifts and have a good home cooked meal. As years passed, my sisters and brothers and I left to get married and have families of our own. After when we gathered for Christmas at my Parents' house, the house seemed smaller because the family was much larger. But the love was still there. Mom and Dad had so much to give. There were more gifts to buy and more food to prepare, but Mother didn't mind. She was full of joy and singing her favorite song, "Christmas Comes But Once A Year". Everyone was invited. If a stranger was passing by, Mother, she would invite them to eat. I shed some tears now when I think of how it used to be. I miss Mother. Christmas of 1988 was the last time we were together as one family.

My Dad Jessel Smith Sr. was born on March 9, 1927. He accepted Christ at a Tent Revival July 30, 1986 and was baptized at the Greater New St. Peter Baptist. He was a tall, medium built and very handsome man. He had a laugh/chuckle that was very unique. He was very smart and very intelligent. He was never educated or attended college. My Dad could add, subtract, multiply and divide without using a calculator. While you were on the calculator, he already had the answer. He was just that good and quick. My Dad could read a blue print and could built a house without one. He was a self taught, self made contractor and he was good at what he did. He built the house we lived in and gave us a home. My Mother was his queen and he was her king. He was a man that loved his eight children and adored all his grandchildren. He was a man who loved God, his church and his pastor. That love reflected in his life.

He was a man that was very good with his hands. He loved to garden and worked around the house and the yard.

He worked hard to make sure his wife and children had what they needed. He made sure we stayed in school and we attend church. His father, Rev. Landry Smith, was a leading pastor in the community. He pastored the Second African Baptist Church. As years passed, I watched this wonderful brilliant man's mind deteriorate. His memory was slowly fading away. My Dad died January 27, 2008. Around Edgard he was known as Rev. and the man in the little white car.

My Nieces Morisa Wells and Trajai Smith wrote a poem when he passed, it reads, "To My Dearest Family."

Although my life has passed away; There are some things I'd like to say. First, I want you all to know, I've made it to my heavenly home. Terry, your mother is as beautiful as the day she left. Though since she's been gone; we've constantly wept. Bum, Boscoe is up here smiling down on you. Knowing and seeing everything you do. Linda, DeDad was welcomed by all with open arms. Monna, the Daddy of all Daddy has me cradled, soft and warm, Keman, boy, I see you in my car. Be careful, watch out for those people; don't cause them any harm. Gail, you've always believe in me, You know I didn't hit those people; they just walk in front of me.

I've made it home. I'm more comfortable and peaceful than I was on earth. So, please don't be unhappy just because my body is being laid in dirt. Remember that I'm with you morning, noon and night. Of course, I've preached a good word and I'm holding a spot for each of you. But the Greatest Daddy of them has all the last word, be assured he'll see you through. He told me your children must invite him in just like everyone else. So my last request, each one of you, get to know Him in order to save yourself and make it in. Because, Tuttie, there is no vacation that you been on, that's greater and more wonderful than our Father Heavenly Home. If God stays the same, I'll see you again. Love and Good-Bye, De-Dad Jessel "Rev" Smith

There were times after Mother died we would gather for Dad's Birthday and we did gather for Christmas 2007. That was the last time that I remember that we were together as a family. That is the last Christmas we had with our Dad. Today, I just say a prayer at Holidays. Since the passing of my Dad and Mother, my family have always made me feel like an outcast. It was that way long time before, but when Mother was around, I would never miss a family gathering. I still love them, despite of how they make me feel. Except for my siblings, Monna Green and Donald Smith, they do call and visit once in a while.

What hurt me the most is that when my parents passed, my siblings took everything. I was the one who was there the most and I am the one that ended with nothing. That hurt! No one thought that I wanted or deserved something. Who is Gail? To them, nobody. Why do they treat me this way? I am their sibling, but you would never know it. Still I love them and pray for them. Can you see stress? I Do Now!

Other major loss in my life that left me feeling stress is the loss of my brother/sibling Jessel "Bosco" Smith. Bosco died February 8, 2000. I always felt my family treated me in a way that I was less than them, but I still love them and we are still a family. My brother, Bosco was a fun loving person at heart. He always had a smile, a joke or a story to tell you. If was hard to tell if he was serious, upset or hurting. His words were "I am alright." He has two beautiful children, Jessel III and Trajai Smith. I was enraged, overwhelmed with sadness, lost and mad at the same time. He was my brother. How am I to move on without my brother? I can't really explain the emotion that I was having. I can't explain the grief I was having. For me this was not real, this was not happening. This can not be true. His death really hurt. My emotions were all over the place. I was so stressed out, did not know where I was. There was so much grief and anger that I became ill. I ended up in the hospital to have emergency surgery, hysterectomy, February 20, 2000. I could not stop bleeding since his funeral. Can you feel the stress? I Do Now!

Other loss that affected me is, my brother-in-law, Freddie "Ponnuty" Young. Ponnuty died February 13, 2009. That was my 56 year birthday!!! He was married to my husband's sister, Myrtis Harris Young. He was a loving and caring person. I can still see him playing with his guitar and playing the guitar while his nephews sing. He played the group called The Golden Echoes. He loved and adored his wife. His children Freddie

Young, Jacqueline Sorapuru, Wanda Draten, Barbara Bernard and his grandchildren were his precious gems. He loved to have them around. You could see it in his face and smile. He always made me feel welcome and I loved him.

The passing of my best friends, Donna Lewis Lumar, January 23, 2009, Leora Marie Howard, September 9, 2009 and Beverly Mitchell Lumar, December 10, 2010 also affected me. Donna Lumar was killed when a train hit the car she was riding in. It happened on the track at my house one morning. I was on my way home from work and they were on their way to work. It was a day I will never forget. I was turning down the street when it happened. Imagine how I felt when I was told she was in the car. I was in shock, could not move, did not know if I wanted to scream, cry or what. I was in so much pain. My friend was in that car. I have to live with this and be reminded of that day, every time I cross the railroad track. I stop and look at the spot she died. I cry! Some days I walk to the track and just look, again I cry! Can You See The Stress? I Do Now!

Marie Howard and Beverly Lumar were two friends that would give you the clothes off their back, if you needed it. Every time you talk to them, it was about their Children. They loved those children. They were two friends I could call or visit at anytime and talk. They would listen and you can be sure what ever I said to them, stayed there and whatever they said to me, stayed there. I was at Marie's bedside when she died. It hurt to see her pass. I was hard to let go, to say Goodbye. Marie was married to Junius Howard and the mother of Kimberly, Kelli, Keldrich, Kristen and

Kip Howard and a grandmother. I was at work when Beverly Lumar passed. Beverly is the former wife of my first cousin, Jerry Lumar Sr. and the mother of Jerry Jr, Juanier, Jovani Lumar and Andre Mitchell. When I got the word that she passed, I could not finish my shift. Their loss hurt and I will never forget my friends. Marie and Beverly were my classmates, Class of 1971, Second Ward High School.

They were my friends. Their passing left a void in my heart. They may be gone, but I will never forget them. The loss of a loved one is one of life's most stressful event and can cause a major emotional crisis. When loss takes place, you experience so many emotions, especially when the death is unexpected. You experience denial, shock, anger, sadness, disbelief and etc. It's not easy to cope. The grief affected me physically, emotionally and psychologically . I shed some tears and I still shed tears. It takes time to fully absorb the impact of a loss. You will never stop missing them, but the pain eases after time and allows you to go on. Can you see the stress? I DO NOW!

Matthew 5:4, "Blessed are the one who mourn for they shall be comforted." John 11:25-26, "I am the resurrection and the life, saith the Lord; he that believeth in me though he were dead, yet shall he live; and whosoever liveth and believeth in me shall never die."

One other factor in my life that really affected me is the arrest of my son-in-law. My son-in-law is currently in prison. It was some years back, I know it was the month of August, I just can't remember the year that my husband preached the Usher's Anniversary at our

Church. We were in the Church's kitchen socializing when his cellphone rang. He said we had to leave, emergency. When we got into the car, he told me my son-in-law attacked and try to rape my daughter, not his wife. He was on the run. My daughter was traumatized, hysterical, scared, angry and hurt Thank God she was able to fight him off. My other daughter, his wife was also very much affected by this. This was her sister, her best friend and he is her husband. She did not how to feel or react. She loves her husband. He is the father of her child. Now we were also caught between two daughter. Which one are we to support? Can you imagine what this was doing to the family? Can You See The Stress? I Do Now!!

He was eventually caught and arrested. He went to prison for 3 years. When he was released, he and my daughter were back together. My husband and I accepted him back into the family because of her and her sister also put her feeling aside because of her sister. She loves her sister and they are best friends. Can You See The Stress? I Do Now!!

But I wish it had end there. He was arrested again, August 2009 for eight counts of carnal knowledge of a juvenile and eight counts of contributing to the delinquency of juveniles. He served ten years and was released March 2017. My husband and I spent our life saving for legal fees, trying to help him because of my daughter and grandkids. We love our daughter and grandchildren and do what ever we can for them. We went though a lot because of this. Can You See The Stress? I Do Now! It doesn't end there. Once again he was arrested. March 2018 he was arrested again for two counts of indecent behavior with a juvenile and sexual battery. He is currently in prison for this crime and waiting for his trial. He has put this family through a lot. He needs help, he has a sickness and will continue down this path until he gets help. We have accepted the fact that we can't help him, he has to be willing to help himself. He needs God in his life. Until he learns to accept God and turn to God for help, he will always be burdened down by this illness and spend the rest of his life behinds bar. Can you See The Stress? I Do Now?

Romans 3:23, " We have all done, thought or said bad things, which the Bible calls "sin". The Bible says, "All have sinned and fall short of the glory of God". Romans 6:23, The result of sin is death, spiritual separation from God."

My daughter is a strong, determined women. She is dedicated to her kids. She is now a single mother and a grandmother and is doing great. She has moved on with her life. I am proud of her and proud of the improvements she has made. She is a praying woman, believes in God and knows that no matter what, God Is Still In Control!!

Joshua 1:9, "Be strong and courageous. Do not be afraid; do not be discouraged for the Lord your God is with you wherever you go."

GAIL COMMINIE

## Chapter 5:
## "When I notice a Change"

For years I have been living under stress and never even realized it. I wrote the beginning chapter to high light a better understanding of what lead up to stress that changed my life.

My siblings, my marriage and kids at a young age. I held the depression, tension and stress in.

If you recall early, I wrote about my marriage to my husband. In the beginning it was all good. Then problems began to work its way in. I told you about the years of abuse and having children in between. The abuse went on for years and I lived in silence. Who do you turn to and when you don't know where, when or who?

Money was tight, we were on rent and barely had food to eat on some days. If it wasn't for my Mother-in-Law, Leanne Comminie and Father-in-Law, Joseph Comminie, I don't know what would have happened to my family. My Mother-in-Law was the best in the world. She always say, 'Gail, hang in there, it will get better. My mother-in-law was a God fearing women.

She not only spoke the Word, but she lived the Word. She was to me a example of a Women of God. She not only talked it but she walked it as well. She would always listen and never took side. She would always be honest and let you know if you were wrong. My husband was her son but she never give him right, or took his side, if he was wrong. There is not to many women today like her. I love her and I miss her smile and her words.

My father-in-law always brought groceries and fruits. He spoiled my kids. They were the apple of his eyes. My favorite memory of him is when I was pregnant with JJ. He would take me to Charity Hospital for my treatment. At Charity Hospital, you would be there for hours. He would always take my girls, Tammy and Shantel with him. He would sit in the Burger King across the street with them and they loved it because they got their burgers, fries and ice cream and they were with Grand Pa Joe Joe. He never complained not once. He would just patiently wait. When JJ was born, he said he wanted him name Joseph Comminie III and so it was!

My husband, one day met the Lord and he slowly began to change. It did not all happen over night, but he begin to slowly change.

It was then that my Mom got sick. Someone had to take care of Mother because my Dad needed to work to keep the insurance for her care. I went to my husband and I told him the situation. I was afraid to but I ask if I could stay home and take care of her. He looked at me and I waited for a response and it was not what I expected. He said, "She is your Mother, do what you have to do and I would support you". Not what I expected to hear. For three years Mother was in and out of the hospital. For three years I was there with her. My sister Monna, my brother Donald, My Aunt Eula Johnson, Aunt Margaret Lumar, Aunt Mildred Samuel, Aunt Julia Joseph and Uncle Veno Samuel would make sure I had a way to get back and forth every day. My husband never once complain, my kids never went without and we never had anything turn off. Sure we struggle but God kept us. It was quite a strain on me both mental and physical, but I kept going. Mother needed me. That Christmas, of 1988 Mother went to my Sister Monna Green. Monna is a school teacher and was off the next two week. She decided she was going to take Mother the two weeks, to give me a break and so I could rest. Thank God for my sister. We have a good relationship,

So we gathered at Monna's on Christmas Day. Mother kept telling me and Monna that she was ready to go home. Monna and I kept telling her to stay one more week with Monna and she will go home. But she kept saying she wanted to go home. So we agree, we will bring her back to her house and I would come in the next morning. Little did we know she was talking about her Heavenly Home.

That Morning when I arrived at the house, I went into the room. I reach for Mother's basin for her bath and I heard a voice say, "Put it down, your work is done!". I said to myself, am I losing it. So I put my hand on the basin again and the voice repeated itself. I asked myself, what going on here? I look at Mother and she just smiled and shook her head. So for the third time I picked up the basin and voice got very loud and said, "Put it down, go home, your work is done!" I looked at mother and she just smiled and said to me, "It's okay." I walked out of the room and looked back at Mother. I assumed she went to sleep, but she had died. I tried to go back into the room, but something or some type of presence was blocking the door. So I did not try to go in but decided to go home and not say a word. Why? because the presence that was in the room, instructed me to do so.

My brother. Jessel Jr. ask, "Are you through already", I just told him, Yes! My Dad ask the same question and I said Yes! Could you please bring me home?

I did not have a phone back then, but my neighbor did. I waited for the phone call. It came at 3 pm. I left Mother's at 9 am and it was not until 3 pm when someone called to say your Mother had passed. I had no ill feeling or regrets for taking care of Mother. God knew she was tired and He knew I had did my best.

After Mother died, my life felt empty. I had nothing to do now. I became bored. Sure, I had the kids and my husband, but I needed something else. So I went back to work and school.

Once again the tension in my marriage arise again. I was under so much stress, depressed all the time and found myself crying a lot. I was so tired. I had to find a solution, an answer. I needed something to escape to. Can You See The Stress? I Do Now!

My solution to my problems was to work harder on myself. I decided to better myself through education and a deep desire to serve God. I had to turn things around. I kept saying to my self, Joseph love me, I just have to respect him more, I am to self-righteous and controlling. I need to be more humble and more obedience. But that did not make a difference. I became more quiet, smaller and he became bigger, louder and more demanding, I was hanging on by a tread. I need a miracle, a healing, I needed God to step in and heal this marriage.

I worked at a gas station and attended The River Parish Community College, in Reserve, La. I received a certificate for Introduction to Computer, January1, 1996 and I received my Associate Degree from Medical Career Institute, Metairie, Louisiana, January 24, 1997 for EKG, Phlebotomy, and CNA. I worked at East Jefferson Hospital, Kenner Behavioral Health and Oschner of Kenner.

I was going to school and working, I still had a family and home to take care of full time. I worked mostly night shifts. I was so tired on some days. I was not getting enough rest, eating right or taking care of self. It was all about the $$$. I was putting so much into just getting and forgetting the things that was most important. Can you see the stress building up? I Do Now!

The tension at home was also rising. I never felt appreciated or really loved. Nothing that I do ever seem to please my husband. The constant criticism and complaints. I just kept it all in. Can you see the stress? I DO NOW!

I never had a voice, it was his way or no way. Can you see the stress? I DO NOW!

Children who demand attention, Can you see the

stress? I Do NOW!

House to maintain, laundry to be done, meals to prepare, errands to run, Can you see the stress? I DO NOW!

Where was I in all this? Can you see the stress? I DO NOW!

Of all the people and things I had to take care of, I was no where on the list. I never saw the stress coming or building up. I need God. My tension was becoming overwhelming, but I know God had not abandoned me. Rather, He was drawing me closer to Him. He healed my marriage in time. Things begin to slowly get better. I remember the words of my Mother-in-Law, Leanne Comminie, "Gail, hang in there, It will get better."

May 1, 2018 we celebrated 47 years of marriage. Yes it was rough and I thought of ending it many times. I wanted to give up. Yes, there was a lot of bad days, but there was some good days also. Marriage takes work. It takes sacrifice. It is not easy, but you have to be wiling to work and sacrifice to make it. When I look back at what I went through, I know it was God that kept me, It was God that give me the strength to endure. It was God that kept me from ending it all. Many times I thought to end it all. I thought that death was better than what I was going through. When you cry yourself to sleep every night and wake up crying, you know things were not good. Things had to get better. Can You See The Stress? I Do Now! Now I have a story to tell others.

## Chapter 6:
### "It take Two"

I can't put all the blame on my husband. I have to take some responsibility for myself. I let him rule. I let him be in control. I never spoke up for myself. I had a voice and I never used it. I was afraid, because I let myself be afraid. I was intimated, because I let myself be intimated. I am a very intelligent women and is capable of many things. So why was I afraid?

My husband is a Minister. He accepted Christ as his personal Savior in the town of Geismer, Louisiana and was baptized at the Greater New St. Peter Baptist Church, Rev. Vernon Alexander, May 26, 1976. He became a Deacon. He received his calling to preach the Gospel, August 4, 1984. On March 29, 1897, he received his license. He was ordained by the Central Union Missionary Baptist Association, June 5, 1993. He became the Church's Youth Minister. Together we organized and the directed the Adult Drama Ministry, January 1995. Request for this ministry have gone on throughout the entire tri-parish and New Orleans Area. We also organize a Annual Youth Retreat. We did a lot of work together in the church. While we appeared good together in the Church, we just couldn't get our personal life on track.

Again, I must accept my part in the blame as well. I could of just said, we need to talk and let him know how I was feeling. Keeping quiet about things and holding them in is not always the right answers. Can you see the stress? I DO NOW!

I would sit and listen as my Husband would counsel other, especially, other married couples or couples to get married. I would just think to myself, he has all the answer but he is not applying it to us. That was my chance to speak up. Again, I just kept silence. I knew we had a problem and I chose not to address it. It takes two and it also takes one to lead.

The Church said the Husband is the head of His wife.

Ephesians 5:23, "For the husband is the head of the wife even as Christ is the head of the church, his body, and is himself its Savior."   Ephesians 5:22, "Wives, submit to your own husband ,as to the Lord."

Yes, I agree with that. But does that means, you control and she does not have a voice or opinion? We are suppose to be one body. We are to live united and together. It does mean one person is better than the other. We are to submit to each other with becoming inferior. As a wife and a Believer of the Scripture, I know that I am commanded to "submit" to my husband as I would to Christ and to show him respect and He is to show me respect. As my husband, The Scripture says he is to love me as Christ love the Church; with humility and sacrifice, as caring for his own body. The Scripture says, we as Christian, Husband and Wives must avoid sexual immorality, avoid vulgar language, foolishness, hate, abuse and any other inappropriate behavior.

There were and are things that you can do if you are in an abusive marriage or relationship. So what do you do when a husband or wife blames and won't take responsibility for his or her bad behavior, well, Don't accept blame. Know for certain that you are not at fault/blame for your husband, wife or partner's behavior. No one can cause you to act in a certain way. Your spouse/partner is abusive because he or she chooses to be that way and it is not your fault. Get outside help. There are no harm or shame in asking or seeking help. There are services available for help. Call if you need to. You may not be an expert on how to stop the violence, abuse or may not be strong enough to stand up to your abuser. Admit you need help because you don't know how to stop the abuse. You need some extra strength, Get help from others. You know that if you are sick, you go to the doctor, if you need legal help, you get a lawyer. Well if you need help in a abusive relationship, the police, dial 911, women shelters, domestic help hotline, the Church, is there to help you. Ask for help, please. Don't compromise. You are responsible for taking care of yourself and your children. Stop putting yourself and them in danger. If someone continue to abuse you, leave them or challenge them to change. Challenge them to treat you with respect and to treat you with the love you deserve. Stop the hate and replace it with kindness. When you or your partner take responsibility for his or her behavior then she can move to change their behavior to one that is loving and caring, If that person is not willing to change, then leave. You have a right to be treated respectfully. That abusive behavior is a choice, Don't accept it. If you are the abuser, STOP it.

## CHAPTER 7:
### "WORK IN FRONT, CHURCH STEP BACK"

Luke 12:15, "Then he said to them, "Watch out! Be on guard against all kinds of greed: a man's life does not consist in the abundance of his possession."

I was Baptized, November 1980, at the Greater New St. Peter Baptist Church.

Now I was very active in the Church. I was Director for the Youth Department, under my husband, involved in the Drama Ministry, Vacation Bible School Teacher, Sunday School and Christian Board of Education, Deaconess Board. Slowly my involvement began to lack. As years passed, I found myself working more and spending less time at Church. I know I was lacking, but I needed to and wanted to work. God was beginning to take a back seat in my life. I work mostly because I hated being home. Work was my way of escaping. There was just too much tension there. Instead of facing my problems, I found a way of escaping and that was work. I found myself turning to food. I was over eating. I indulged in food. I was gaining weight and my blood pressure was rising. I was up to 268 lbs. My health was in danger. I was crying all the time. At work, I would go into the bathroom or break room and cry. I was crying at Church, people thought it was because of something said or a song sung at the service. Crying while driving, watching TV, cooking, washing, crying all the time. I put on a great show. I was a great pretender. You could never tell, I was in trouble. I was living a lie!! CAN YOU SEE THE STRESS? I DO NOW!!

I was near my breaking point. I was in serious health danger.

But God have a way of bringing us back into reality and to Him.

When we think we have it all in control and we have all the answers. I was neglecting my Church and my First Love, but I kept going. I was working the night shift at Ochsner Medical Center, Mother Baby Unit. One morning, October 28, 2013, I went to the mail box to mail a letter and set down to write my son, Jamaal and his wife Ranada a note. When I picked up the pen, I could not write or control the pen. I felt a little strange and notice a slur in my speech. I said to myself, "I am having a stroke." I knew the warning signs of a stroke from my medical training. My husband was not home, so I phoned him and tried to explain, but he knew something was wrong. He told me to hang up and he was going to call his cousin, Vivian Chopin, who live next door. Vivian came and immediately call the ambulance and call my husband back and phone his sister Myrtis Young. My husband met the ambulance and they told him, I was having a stroke and there is a three hour window to get help. Not sure of how much time had passed, I was flown by helicopter to Ochsner, Main Campus, New Orleans, Louisiana. I was given TPA, tissue plasminogen activator. This drug must be given immediately. Every passing minute counts.

I was in ICU for a few days. While I was in the hospital, I kept asking, "Why me, Lord?" I was now in a life changing situation. I never thought this would happen to me. I was having a real struggle over this. Me, a stroke. I am a very busy person, with Church, home and the community. This can't be happening. I am glad I recognized the signs of a stroke and acted immediately. It saved my life and from long term difficulty.

God allowed things to happen, but that doesn't means He necessarily caused it. There are many things that happen to us that we may never understand on this side of Heaven and we can only turn to God and trust Him to bring us out of this. Sometimes God allowed bad things to happen, so He could get us in a place where He has our full and undivided attention. Sometimes He need to talk to us and we need to listen. The real question we need to ask when sickness comes or things go wrong, isn't why it happen, but how God wants us to responds. We should Thank God for sparing our lives.

1 Thessalonians 5:18, "Give thanks in all circumstances, for this is God's will for you in Christ Jesus."

God doesn't want us to spend our time thinking about the past or complaining about things we can't do anything about. Complaining just makes you more miserable and more stressed and more depressed. Ask God to help you and to help you accept the situation and show you how you can serve Him in the place you are now. None of us want to go through trials or to be tested by God. Many of you have been through some level of trials or hardship or experience some level of pain at some time in your life. Not only the Christians go through hardship and experience pain. But non-Christian are also tested and go through trials, even if they don't believe in God or know Jesus Christ. God put us through things to refine us.

Zachariah 13:9, 'And I will bring the third part through the fire, and will refine them as silver id refined, and will try them as gold is tried; they shall call on my name, and I will hear them; I will say, it is my people; and they say, The Lord is my God.".

Things will happen in our lives that we don't understand so that he may refine or transfer us into the person he wants us to be. We will have financial problem, hunger and sickness so that we may seek Him and trust Him. He put us through things to prove to prove to Satan and the world that we are a child of God.

1 Peter 1:7, "That the trial of our faith, being much more precious than gold that perisheth though it be tried with fire, might be found unto praise and honour and glory at the appearing of Jesus Christ;".

Read the story of Job. Satan accused Job of only serving God because he put a hedge of protection around him. He puts us through trials to help us grow.

Roman 8:28, "And we know that in all things God works for the good of these who love him, who have been called according to his purpose."

He put us through trials to test you and to let you know He is God and that you may want to know more of Him.

Job 42:5, "I had only heard about you before, but now I have seen you with my own eyes."

After my stroke, it was hard. I felt sorry for me. Then I had a second stroke, December 15, 2013. This time I was in the wheel chair and had difficulty speaking. I now depending on others for help. I hated this. I have always been independent. I have always on the go. I did my own thing. Now I had to wait for someone to help me. I was so depressed. Then one day, my Cousin Dornell Herbert came by to see me. I was surprised, because this was the first time he ever visit or came to my home. He told me his story. He had a stroke and made a recovery. He wanted to share his testimony of how God brought him through.

Psalm 6:6, "Come and listen, all you who fear God, and I will tell you what he did for me."

I was stunned. He had a stroke, this man standing here in my living room, talking to me. I could not believe it! He prayed with me and said "Trust God", He will come through. When He left, I was still stunned. I look up toward Heaven and said, "God, if you did it for Him, you can do it for me."

Daniel 4:2, "I want you all to know about the miraculous signs and wonders the Most High God has performed for me."

I was still depressed, but I decided I was going to beat this with God's help. So I begin speech therapy, occupation therapy and physical. It was long and hard but I was determined. Slowly, I began to get better and out of the wheelchair and walking with a cane. My speech, memory and thought process was still slow, but this is something I have to live with. I suffer a third stroke, TIA on January 9, 2014. A minor set back.

My husband has been great and very supportive. He has made a remarkable change.

Ezekiel 36:6, :And I will give you a new heart, and a new spirit I will put within you. And I will remove the heart of stone from your flesh and give you a heart of flesh."

I don't know if the stroke scared him. When he was told by the ambulance driver, that I had to be flown to the hospital because time was critical, it did something to him. I was told, he broke down and cried. He was by my bedside everyday I was in the hospital. My husband has been my caregiver, my supporter and has been there for me since day one of my stroke. He has been by my side everyday. He was pushing me in the wheel chair, putting me in and out of the tube, helping me dress, preparing meals, taking care of the house, running errands, making sure I took meds. He was at my side every step of the way. Illness has a way of bringing people together. Illness has a way of making you see what you have and what you could lose. Illness makes you realize just what that person really means to you. I had to have out patient therapy, he brought me and stayed until I was done. If I wanted something, he made sure I got it. We talk for hours about anything and everything. It was like we are in love again. We grew closer and stronger. My stroke has change him, made my marriage stronger and we are both better person because of it. God has a way of doing things. I thank God everyday for bringing us closer together. I never thought this would ever happen. God has healed our marriage and brought us closer together when I needed him the most. After all these years I love him more today than yesterday. We have been married 47 years on May 1, 2018. Things have not always been easy, but it was worth fighting for. With the help of God, we stuck it out. We are better people and a better couple. Yes, we have our moments, but now we disagree in a new way. I have a voice and I am now free to express my self.

To my husband I say, I love you. You are my best friend. Those 47 yeas have been worth it. Yes, we fought, but we stayed together. Yes, there were some difficulties, but we stayed together, Yes, there were some stressful moments, but we stayed together. Yes, there were times I felt like giving up and you did to, but we stayed together. We knew deep down inside, we had something worth staying for and fighting for. The things we went through have strengthened us. I am not saying all is perfect. We have our good days and our bad days. But now I am no longer afraid, I am no longer ashamed, I no longer afraid of what people are saying or will find out. I have a voice now. I can express myself when we disagree and my opinion counts. Yes, He is the head of the wife, according to Ephesiana 5: 22. I am proud that he is head.

God has blessed us in so many ways. We have four beautiful children together, Tammy Gullage, Shantel Octave, JJ Comminie, Jamaal Comminie and two beautiful daughter-in-laws, Ranada Comminie, Mtisa

Comminie and one-son-in-law, Shannon Octave Sr. We have eleven grandchildren, Anastasia, Leonard Jr., and Larenz Gullage, Shannon Jr. and Shayler Octave, Jeremiah , Jamaal Jr., Ja'Quan Comminie, Randall and Syan Clark, Danasha Harris. Three great grand children, Jaceon and Jason Debery and Aubrie Gullage. God has truly Bless Us.

I just want you to know you are truly a great husband, father and friend. After 47 years, I love you more after each passing day. Yes, we have been through so much, but we have fought the battles together and we are together and stronger. You are a Man of God and I am proud to stand by your side as you wife and partner. I love You.

Ephesians 4:2-3, 'Be completely humble and gentle: Be patient, bearing with one another in love. Make every effort to keep the unity of the spirit through the bond of peace." Ephesians 4:32, " And be kind to one another, tenderhearted, forgiving one another, even as God in Christ forgave you." "Rev Joseph Comminie Jr."

## Chapter 8: "After My Stroke"

Psalm 107:20, "He sent out his word and healed them, and delivered them from their destruction."

Psalm 41:3, "The Lord sustains him on his sickbed; in his illness you restore him to full health."

After my stroke there are still some things that happened in my life that were stressful. But this time I have learned how to cope. There is still the same issue with my siblings. They still treat me like a outsider. I don't live in or have the big house they have, but live in a house and my house is a home. I don't drive the big car like them, but I have a car. When they gather for holidays, they invite me, but always ask me to bring drink. Why? Because to them I can't cook or not clean enough for them. News…I am a great cook, better then they think and better then them. My house in immaculate/clean and I am clean. I am treated like I am the black sheep. I always stay home with my family or join my in-laws for theirs. There I am always welcome and with open arms. CAN YOU SEE THE STRESS? YES, I Do!!

God gave us sibling to provide support when life goes haywire. God gave us sibling to pray for one another. God gave us sibling for encouragement. God gave us sibling so that we will not be alone.

Seeing me seems to annoy them. I am a distraction and a disappointment.

**Can You See The Stress? Yes, I Do!!**

My sister, Monna Green and my little brother, Donald Smith, I must admit do call me now and then, even if just to say Hi. They do visit now and then, even if It's not long. My niece Morisa Wells, Monna's daughter is like a daughter to me. That child worry to much and always call to check on her Auntie. During my strokes, they did come by and offer support to me and my husband. I love them and thank them for that.

I loss my nine year old niece, Jayla Ashawn Smith, September 22, 2016. She was born a gift from God to my nephew, Jessel Smith II and Keyoka Joseph. She was gifted and loved. She loved doing care package for the homeless using her donations from National Lemonade Day. She was little girl, with a immaculate smile and a big heart. Everybody loved Jayla. She leave behind her little sister Kaysha Smith. Even though I only knew her for a little while, she touched my heart, and is my inspiration on how we much to show love. Can You See The Stress? Yes, I Do, Now!

While walking in the yard, November 22, 2016, I fell. Suddenly I lost my balance and my both of my legs went out. The fall left me with some bruises and I knocked out my tooth. I was bleeding from the lip and the mouth. My neighbor Lester Chopin is always in his yard doing something. That day he was nowhere to be found. I had to crawl to my back door step to get up.

My daughter, Tammy Lynette Gullage, was admitted to the hospital with a stroke on January 7, 2017. I was so worried about Tammy, my first born. She have been through a lot and now this. Could you imagine what it like to see your child go through this, especially when you been through it. I was concern about her three children who love and depend so much on Mother. I was sitting on her bed, feeling stressful and terrified. I was feeling helpless. There was nothing I could do to change what has happen. CAN YOU SEE THE STRESS? Yes, I Do Now!! I prayed to God, "Please help, heal, my child."

Psalm 23:1-3, The Lord is my shepherd; I have everything I need. He lets me rest in fields of green grass and leads me to quiet ponds of fresh water He gives me new strength. He guides me in the right paths as he has promised."

I am so happy to say she did recover and was only left with some minor lasting effects.

While sitting on Tammy's bed at the hospital, I was not feeling well. I was really weak, appetite was poor and very nausea. My husband and I decided to leave and would be back in the morning. While walking in the hospital hallways, I had to hold on to the walls because I was just that weak. I didn't think I would make to the truck. I just barely made it. My husband stop for gas and I open up the door because I felt like I wanted to vomit. I did, but it was blood and a lot. I call my husband over to see and I kept vomiting blood. He wanted to go back to the hospital, but I said no, take me home. All the way home from Kenner to Edgard, I was vomiting blood. By the time I got home, I was very weak from vomiting and losing blood. I could not even take my clothes off or barely focus. My husband called 911 and I was taken to the nearest hospital, St. James Hospital in Lutcher, Louisiana. The Emergency Room Doctor there told me that all he could do was stabilize me and transfer me to Ochsner Baptist in New Orleans, Louisiana. I appreciate him being honest with me. He had never treated this before. So I was given blood transfusion and transfer. That was January 8, 2017. I was admitted to ICU at Oschner Baptist and was told I needed surgery. I suffered a 'Mallory Weiss Tear' which is a tear to the lower esophagus. My other health issues are high blood pressure, cholesterol, anemia, GERD, osteoarthritis of the right knee, right shoulder rotator cuff, obesity and aphasia which is loss of language or speech, may not be able to explain or understand things because the part of the brain that control the language was destroy due to the stroke. I have had three surgery where the doctor had to go in and open up my esophagus so I could swallow. I am still at risk for another stroke which could be serious. Can You See The Stress? Yes, I Do Now!

John 16:33, "I have said these things to you, that in me you may have peace. In the world you will have tribulation. But take heart; I have overcome the world.'"

My grandson, JaQuan Joseph Comminie, was born September 7, 2017 at OakBend Medical Center, Houston, Texas. He weigh 8lbs and 6 oz. Right after his birth, he was having difficulty breathing and was not getting enough oxygen.  He was air lifted to Houston Methodist Hospital and was admitted to ICU.  He was in very critical condition.   He was diagnosed with Hypoplastic Left Heart Syndrome (HLHS) which is a birth defect that affects the normal blood flow through the heart.  This is one type of congenital heart defect.  On September 11, 2017 just four days old, he had open heart surgery.  On March 22, 2018 he under went his second open heart surgery.

"Isaiah 41:10, "So do not fear, for I am with you; do not be dismayed, for I am your God.  I will strength you and help you ; I will uphold you with my righteous right hand."

I was hurting so bad for my grandchild. I could not find the words to pray.  I just sit in silence and hope that God understand.  I wanted to pray but I couldn't.  I know that God hears our hearts. My heart is breaking for my child and his child and my grandchild,  I don't understand why God would let this happen to a baby.  While in the hospital, I saw so many other sick babies and my heart went out to them and their family.  I was not the only one suffering.  In silence I said a prayer and I know that God heard me.

My mind went to, Isaiah 55:8-10 "Your ways are higher than my ways. Your thoughts are higher than my thoughts.'"

Jeremiah 30"17, But I  will restore you to health and heal your wounds; declare the LORD"

When you are  face with health problems, bad news, relationship problem, The Word of God is your help.  Don't Give Up!  Talk to GOD!!

Baby Ja'Quan is doing fine now and his next surgery should be when he is five year old.

I loss my brother-in-law, Charles "Coba" Harris on Christmas day, December 25, 2017. Suddenly he was gone. It caught us by surprise. This will be a Christmas I will always remember and will remember ever Christmas after. He was the one who visit everybody. He would come by everyday to check on me and see if I need anything. All of the children loved their Uncle Bubba and Uncle Bubba spoil them all and had nickname for all of them. I miss him and still look for his knock at the door. Can You See The Stress? Yes, I Do Now?

There is the stress of finance/money. Before my stroke, I was bringing a pretty good paycheck. We were doing okay. The bills were being paid, food on the table and we could spurge every now and then. I was working so much, that I was neglecting the things that matter. That is my God and Church. They were beginning to take a back seat.

God should always be first. He don't want to be last in your life. He has a way of bringing us back to Him. Now we are having financial problem. At first I was on Disability, but now we are on Social Security. Making ends meet is rough. We hardly have any money left to finish the month. Paying the bills and keeping food on the table is a challenge. I am on medications and so is my husband. Thank god, we have children who are able to help us out. Can You See The Stress? Yes, I Do Now! I am waiting for a break through. I know that God know what we are going through. He will come to our aid. I am waiting patiently.

There is so much stress, tension and worry when it comes to our children in the school today. Never have I ever seem or heard of so much destruction and hate. School used to be the safest place we could send our children.

2 Timothy 3:1-4, "This know also, that in the last days perilous times shall come, For men shall be lovers of their own selves, covetous, boasters, proud, blasphemers, disobedient to parents, unthankful, fierce, despisers of those that are good , Traitors, heady, high minded, lovers of pleasure more than lovers of God."

How are we to respond to all this evil today in our school?

School shootings have been making the headlines. Our world is in mourning as school violence increase and has become a part of our lives. Why is there is so much violence and killing among our young people? Why is there so much rapes, fights, robberies, killing? The Bible tells us about a time in history that these kinds of violence will be committed by children all over the world. The Bible speaks of a generation of youth who will be a curse to their parents and others, Can You See The Stress? Yes ,I do?

Isaiah 1:4, "Ah sinful nation, a people laden with iniquity, a seed of evildoers, children that are corrupters; they have forsaken the LORD, they have provoked the Holy One of Israel unto anger, they are gone away backward."

We as parents try to raise our children correctly, in the way God has instructed us to, yet they still are rebellious. We have to continue praying for them, we as parents have to believe that faith and prayer will bring them back to us. Bring them back to what we have taught them. Not all our children are evil, bad, but our children are coming under evil influences in our society which has become a way of death and corruption. Why is there so much violence among our young people. Can you see the stress? Yes, I can!

What can we expect when our TV shows, the music, the video games are filled with violence, sex and murder. Have you ever listened to the music your child listen to? I am a grandmother of eight boys, so I have. Their music consists of suicide, murder, witchcraft and sex. Those so-called artists/musicians are encouraging our children to rebel against their parents, and authorities. I have watched the video games they play, again violence and murder. Parents be on guard, pay attention to what your child has access to. Our children has cellphones and no limitation or restriction to how they are being used. Children learn what they see and hear. The mind is fill with all kinds of evil. Satan is tempting them to act out these things. Some of those children committing these acts of violence has mental issue. Those mental issue is brought on by what is put into their minds. Our society, our world has become obsess with guns and war. Can you see the stress? Yes, I can!

Mark 4:24a, "And he (Jesus) said unto the, Take heed what ye hear."

Prayer in the school has been abandoned but we can teach our children to still pray in silence, to pray at home before going to school. Just pray!!! We as parents have become lacking in our Christian involvement and the things of God. We would rather go to a game, then to Church or prayer meeting. We are more involved in our jobs, our entertainments and other things then going to Church or Bible Class. We have to pray for our children and teach them to pray.

My daughter, Shantel Octave and my sister Monna Green are school teachers. I pray for them and the school everyday. We must Pray!!!

1 Timothy 2:1, "I exhort therefore, that, first of all, supplications, prayer, intercessions, and giving of thanks, be made for all men; For kings, and for all that are in authority; that we may lead a quiet and peaceable life in all godliness and honesty. For this is good and acceptable in the sight of God our Saviour."

## Gail Comminie

# Chapter 9:
## "Coping With Stress"

Psalm 55:22, "Cast your burden on the Lord, and he will sustain you; he will never permit the righteous to be moved."

I can still see the stress, but now I know how to cope. I am on medication, exercise every day, I have lost 103 lb. I was at 268 lb. now I am 165 lb. I am eating right and watching my diet. Coping with stress is not easy, because we live in a stressful world. Stress is how we act physical, mentally and emotionally to things around us. When the people and the world ask more of us than we can give, it is stressful. It is a natural part of life. It becomes harmful when we can't cope. The least thing can stress us out. You can forget to turn off the TV, that will stress you. A major thing like a death off a love one will stress you. A rude/unfriendly/hateful neighbor will stress you. Trust me I know all about that. The Holidays can stress you out. Family visit can stress you out. What to wear can stress you out. What am I going to cook can stress you out. Grandchildren and Children can stress you out. A divorce can stress you out. There are many more thing

I am sure can stress you out. There are many things in life that happen that you can't do anything about. Sometimes you just have to accept things for what they are and move on. There are things that will happen that is behind our control. There are times we might try to fix a problem, only to make it work. We have to learn to just pray and wait on God. Try God and I can testify He will work it out. Just Give it over to the Lord and He will work it out.

Not all stress causes stroke, but having a stroke or someone close to you having a stroke can be very overwhelming. The effect of a stroke can be death, physical impairment and mental issue. It can be serious physical, emotional, social and financial. It is serious for all involved , the person with the stroke, the caregiver and the family.

We all react to stress differently. Recognizing how we act under stressful situations is the first step in gaining control over our feeling of being stress and anxiety.

What are some of the sign of stress? The signs are high blood pressure, headaches, indigestion, stomach pain, change in bowel, chest pain, loss of appetite or eating to much, not getting enough sleep, allergies, loss of sexual desire, your emotion runs high and low, fatigue, aches and pain, always tired and loss of energy.

Mental signs can be depression, poor motivation, smoking or drinking too much,  poor motivation, can't finish a task, don't want to socialize, not being able to plan your day or plan a schedule, poor memory, can't concentrate, anxiety, short temper, and very impulsive behavior.

To cope with stress, change your environment, I mean your living situation or job if you have to. Living in a abusive situation or a unhealthy environment can be stressful. Going to work everyday on a job you hate, can be stressful.

Reduce stress or cope with stress by Talking to someone one you trust. Don't do like I did by bottle things up. Talk! Talk! Talk!

Learn to relax, Medicate or take up yoga. Or just go for or walk or to the beach. Take some time out and enjoy yourself. Try to look at the whole picture, not just the problem and get someone you trust opinion. Learn to take responsible for your own feelings. Let it out. Don't keep it in. GIRL scream and cry as loud and as you can. Make sure no one hears you, but Girl scream and cry, let it out. Change your diet and exercise. Say No, and mean it. Don't let yourself be pressured and don't take on too much, no more then you can handle. Know your strength and your weakness. Learn to accept what you can't change and change what you can. Smile more and Laugh more. Laughter reduces stress and tension. And most important thing to do is "Try GOD!!!"

Jeremiah 30:17, 'but I will restore you to health and heal your wounds; declares the lord.'

## Gail Comminie

# Chapter 10:
## "Faith in Despair"

Proverbs 16:9, "The heart of man plans his way, but the Lord establish his steps,"

Have you ever felt like you never "Made a Prayer?" Have you ever ask yourself "Where is God?" There are times, moments in my life when I have asked myself those question. It is not that I don't know or trust God. I felt that way because sometimes I feel all alone. Things are rough. Money is tight or none at all. Bills are due and I don't have the finance to pay them. I am feeling so bad at times that I feel like this is it. There are time I almost stop praying. It seems like every time I pray, God says, NO!. Why is it so difficult? I look around I see people prosper that don't go to Church or believe. I say "This is not fair, God". Why was I wasting my time, energy or emotion praying to God and God keep saying No!. I wanted to believe that God was saying No, because this was not my time.

Maybe God is answering my prayer. I have to accept, It is God's will not my will" God is saying No because it it is not the right time. God is saying I will move the obstacle when I change my attitude and not complaining so much. Some time I have to learn to wait. I serve an on-time God. He may not come when I want Him but He is on time. God did not answer my prayer because what I though was the best for me wasn't the best for me. You can't hurry God, you can't manipulate God, you can't fool God, you can't have it your way. God is not Burger King. I have to learn to relax and learn to trust God. God is on my side. God only wants the best for me. There is nobody other than God who wants to see me achieve my goals and my dreams. God leads me and He guide me in all truth. I learn to pray, "God, not my will, but your will be done." God will open up the right door and God will close the wrong door. I have to stay open to His direction and follow Him. Proverb, 3:6, In all your ways acknowledge Him and He shall direct your path." So I thank God, that He do not let me have my way. I Thank God that He knows what best for me. I thank God that He is so merciful and He do not let me have my way. I have learn that when God does not answer my prayer, it is because God is protecting me. There may be danger ahead and He is keeping me from harm's way. I have learned when He does not answer my prayer, it is not the right time, be patient, God has something better for me. God knows what is best for me. God can see the future. Every time I wanted to let go, God held me. Through all my sickness, trials and trouble, God was and is there. The battle is not mine, it's the Lord's.

    I have to trust God. God does answer my prayer, but on His time. God has me in His hand. When the time comes, God will open doors for me, that no man can shut. There is nothing too hard for my God. There are no enemies too powerful for my God. My God has the power to turn any situation around. Yes God is there. He is there all the time. I know that when I trust God with my life, I can trust Him with the choices I make and the decision I make, God will lead me to the right choice to the way that is best for me.

Psalm 86:11a, "Teach me your way, or Lord; I will walk in your truth."

My God will never leave me or forsake me.

## Gail Comminie

## Chapter 11:
### "My Support Team"

Ruth 1:8, And may the Lord reward you for your kindness..."

I would like to thank those who have been supportive of me during my strokes and other illness. It has not been easy, but I had and have God on my side. God has put some very important and loving people in my life. He knows just what I need and when I need. My husband Rev. Comminie was and is my biggest supporter. He has stood by me all the way and he is encouraging me on. Things were rough in the beginning but we are getting there.

My children, I don't know what I would do without them. Not a day goes by that they do not call. It is always, Mom are you alright and do you or Dad need anything. I raise some wonderful, God fearing children. They love their Mother and Father and love each other. There is no segregation or separation between them. They treat and respect each other as equal and are there for each other. I have told them, if one don't have and you do, give it to them. If your brother or sister is in need, give them. Always keep in touch and make yourself available to each other. You are brothers and sisters.

My Church members, Rev. Vernon Sr. and Yvonne Alexander, Rev. Joseph and Gail Hilaire, Zelda Dukes, Lovenia Ross, Carol Young, Laura Howard, George and Brenilla Dunmiles, Fabolia Lewis, Mildred Samuel, Ronda Young, Late Claude Gordon. Vivian Chopin, Audrey Valentine, Linda Narcisse, Gloria Mae Howard, Shelia Jones. Alvin and Jessica Narcisse, Valarie Francis. Also Rev. Clearence Mollaire, pastor of Second African Baptist Church, Donell Herbert. Rev. Marc Nelson and Lynelle and the Greater Woodville Baptist Church. Rev. Roland Scott. Your love, your calls, your visits, your gifts, your prayers will always be appreciated.

My cousins, Stella Matthew, Colette Boudoin, Bonnie Grows, Christine Barnes, Gloria Brignac.

My sibling, Monna Green and Donald Smith.

My in-laws, Harold Comminie, Ronald Comminie, Pamela Comminie, Myrtis Young, Dorethia Harris, Shelton Valentine, Sterling Harris, Josie Harris, The Late Charles Harris. My in-laws have always treated me with kindest. They have always made me feel as part of the family. I forget some times that I am related by marriage. They are most loving, giving and kindness people I know.

My Sister-in -Law Brenda Valentine is more of a sister to me than a sister-in-law. She was in my wedding. She had the biggest smile. She is my best friend. I can called her anytime and talk. We can talk about anything and everything. If we disagree, we will take a break, but not a long one...it's just time out She gives me great advice and she is honest. She is just a amazing sister-in-law. A amazing person. Brenda, I love you and Thanks for being my sister-in-law/MY SISTER!

There is a poem, my favorite that I like to read and have a photo of it on my wall
"FOOTPRINTS IN THE SAND"
One Night I dreamed a dream
As I was walking along the beach with my Lord,
Across the dark sky flashed scene from my life.
For each scene, I noticed two sets of footprints in the sand,
One belonging to me and one to my Lord.
After the last scene of my life flash before me,
I looked back at the footprints in the sand.
I noticed that at many times along the path of my life, especially at the very lowest and saddest times, there was only one set of footprints.
This really trouble me, so I ask the Lord about it.
"Lord, you said once I decided to follow you, You'd walk with me all the way.
But I noticed that during the saddest and troublesome times of my life, there was only one set of footprints.
I don't understand why, when I needed You the most, you would leave me."
He whispered, "My precious child, I love you and will never leave you.
Never, ever, during your trials and testing.
When you saw only one set of footprints, 'It was then I carried you."
*******************************████████

Isaiah 38:16-17, 'you restored me to health and let me live. Surely it was for my benefit that I suffered such anguish. In your love you kept me from the pit of destruction; you have put all my sins behind your back.'

Special thanks to my husband Rev. Joseph Commine Jr. who encouraged me to write about my trials and recovery.

Special thanks to my Uncle Ronald Samuel who has always believe in my talents and have encouraged me to pursue my dream.

Special thanks to my children and family who said, "I could do it"

**TO GOD BE THE GLORY FOR THE THINGS HE HAS DONE…AMEN!**

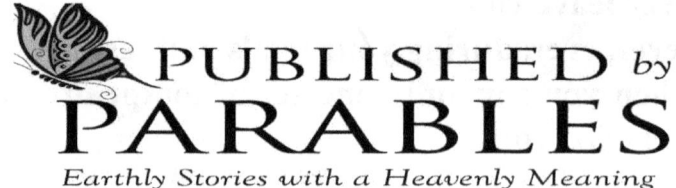

www.ingramcontent.com/pod-product-compliance
Lightning Source LLC
Chambersburg PA
CBHW060033040426
42333CB00042B/2410